Wellness of Life

Bless you !

♡ Angela

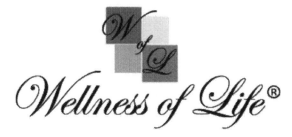

WHOLE BODY WELLNESS WITH EASE

Wellness of Life®
5120 J. Street #G
Sacramento, CA 95819

Online ordering:
www.wellnessoflifeproducts.com
Email: wellnessoflife@gmail.com
Clinic: www.wellnessoflife.com

Phone Number (916) 905-7743

Angela Harris Studies, Research and Entrepreneurship
1991-2005, currently Wellness of Life Clinic™ 2005, currently
Angela Harris Research and Creative Intellectual Property
1999-2020, currently Quotes, Affirmations, Titles by Angela
Harris

Photographs by Shoop's Photography

Book Cover and Design by Tywebbin Creations
Medical Images Photo Stock
Images Isabel Gonzalez

Published by Everything with Love™
Publisher Angela Harris
5120 J.Street
Sacramento, CA 95819

Published in the United States of America
Library of Congress Data available upon request
ISBN: 978-0-578-64378-6

DEDICATION

To my creator, God my hero, whom I look up to. Holy Spirit, thank you for your guidance, counsel, comfort, and most importantly, the spirit of love.

*To my family. My two children and granddaughter, who I look forward to and what my labor of love provides for them. Blessings to my grandparents for their love and acceptance. To family members...I want to say thank you and I'm truly grateful for how they contributed, supported and shared the vision, **Wellness of Life** with me. Bless you for training me for the world, your spoken words, and silent thoughts that helped my heartfelt moments of affirming who I am designed to be in order to contribute to the world.*

To all my clients, truly thankful and grateful for the connection of community.

And to all the astonishing angels throughout the course of my life: I could not have done it without all of you.

I Love You!

Contents

ACKNOWLEDGEMENT

I would like to express my heart of love and appreciation to family, co-laborers, friends, staff, amazing teachers, mentors, and all the divine opportunities to live a life full of blessings, lessons, teachable moments, and reciprocal encouragement that has affirmed my journey, education, and credentials. I would not be the mom, holistic practitioner, entrepreneur, and writer I am today.

Thank You!

INTRODUCTION

Get ready for a holistically, clear insight, a pure connection of articulation on how we have been given all that we need in order for the whole body to potentially heal. Whole Body Health and Wellness with Ease will not focus on the disease, instead we will pay attention to the cause.

The Wellness of Life mission is to provide holistic wellness coaching, substantial services, resources and tools to transition and transform your current healthcare into embracing self-care and believing in self-compassion.

Our desire is to help you turn toward a state of wellbeing. Helping individuals by connecting, communicating and creating a wellness strategy custom made for each individual.

We will discuss cleansing, elimination (releasing) and restoration, in order to give the whole body the opportunity to rebuild itself naturally. This is alignment! My belief in alignment is simply living

Wellness of Life. A relationship between Wellness of Life and our clients consistently committed to addressing the cause and aligning with whole body health and wellness with ease. A series of profound adjustments using wholehearted conversations and efficient proper resources to transition effectively into potential healing. Yes, in that order.

Holistic is a whole picture of all aspects of the individual for assessment to determine what is needed at the present moment in time. We are individuals first. Our families, friendships, occupations and social lives are made up of individuals. As an individual we contribute to all of the above.

Each individual has a gift, talent, skill, and ability destined for life's existence or preoccupied by comparison and compromising. Our bodies know the layers of emotions, the mental stress of the mind, the collection of stored sensory information from the brain, and the heart of the whole person.

Anatomy and physiology show us how we are well made in complete fullness. The capacity of true fulfillment internally. What you see, what you intake into your body, what you tell yourself, and what you believe matters. This is why the relief of releasing is so rewarding.

To share something is to give a portion. My pure intention in writing this book is to supersede sharing and to write with whole fullness. Gently with love and kindness ask yourself, What are you full of? Welcome this question with Ease... If you cannot answer the question right now. Know that self-care requires self-compassion.

To The Reader

Through reading this book, a connection to the information and internal questions provided will help you self-assess, write, see your answers, and by the end of this book you will hopefully and faithfully move forward in creating an individualized strategy through wellness coaching to Live Wellness "of" Life. Over 15 years. Ago. I chose to use the word "of" because it means to "be it,"... "for" is to "support it" and "to" is to "motion to approach it." Let's be it!

Moment of Wisdom

God is Faithful and during opposition and opportunity in our lives the Universe is asking... Are you ready to grow? We have many choices, I made a decision to say YES! And I Trusted God.

Everything with Love,
Angela

CHAPTER 1

Internal Footprint

Everything in your lifetime influences your internal ecosystem leaving different footprints. No matter what the impression was, or is, you have a daily obligation to ask yourself what do you want those footprints to exist as internally before it shows up externally in your life?

Getting to know yourself internally is out of this world astonishing. I believe in whole body health and wellness with ease not disease. No pressure. Why should we add additional stress on the body with an unrealistic approach? We must consider all things in our lives that we have to experience, endure and embrace in order to survive as an individual.

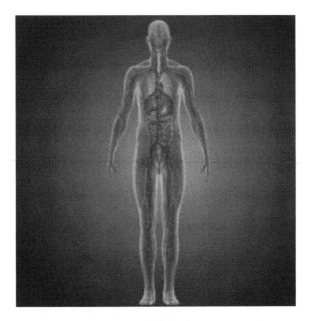

Life is existence and the life cycle is a series of stages through which an individual is exposed to people, cultures, environments, and products moving through one's life until completion occurs during this lifetime.

Each individual's contribution to the world is significant. Through togetherness we can share the differences to teach and learn from each other, creating inspiration and encouragement to improve ourselves, family, friends, coworkers, social environments and community.

What do you believe your contribution to your family, friends, and community is?

Does your reasonable service make a positive difference?

Do you know your difference?

We are purposefully different, intentionally.

~ Wellness of Life

WRITING EXERCISE FOR YOU

Choose three words to describe how you feel in this moment about your health and wellness internally.

Choose three words to describe how you see yourself in this moment physically externally.

> *Life is existence, love is everlasting.*
> *In our existence, share love!*
> ~ Wellness of Life

CHAPTER 2

The Human Body

The human body has eleven distinct systems. Here is a basic straightforward description of each system:

DIGESTIVE SYSTEM – THE POWER

The powerful digestive system provides nutrients and energy to the whole body, allowing the body to function properly. Seventy percent of our immune system is located in the large intestines (colon) and ninety percent of our neurotransmitters. Neurotransmitters communicate information to the brain, and the brain informs the whole body to process regulating mood and cognition. Chemicals produced and released in our Gut is endorphins, serotonin, dopamine, glutamate, norepinephrine, epinephrine, and GABA (gamma-aminobutyric acid).

CIRCULATORY SYSTEM – THE FLOW

This system allows blood to circulate and transports nutrients to and from cells in order to provide nourishment and promote oxygen throughout the whole body. Helping to manage and maintain homeostasis.

ENDOCRINE SYSTEM – THE REGULATOR

The endocrine system regulates glands, hormones, metabolism, growth and sensory organs.

INTEGUMENTARY SYSTEM – THE MAINTAINER

This system is a barrier to protect and support other systems. Consisting of skin, hair, nails, glands and nerves.

LYMPHATIC SYSTEM –THE FILTERATOR

This second part of the circulatory system that traps and destroys bacteria and foreign substances.

MUSCULAR SYSTEM – THE MOTIVATOR

The muscular system creates motion and movement for all actions and functions of the body.

NERVOUS SYSTEM – THE INFORMER

The nervous system communicates and coordinates the information and responses throughout the whole body.

REPRODUCTIVE SYSTEM – THE REPRODUCER

The reproductive system manages the procreation of life, reproduction, through existing life.

RESPIRATORY SYSTEM – THE BREATHER

The respiratory system purifies what we breathe to protect and benefit the body. The body's cells need a continuous supply of oxygen for all the chemical changes that take place in a cell or an organism to produce energy needed for life.

SKELETAL SYSTEM – THE PROTECTOR

This system provides structural support to protect delicate internal organs and supplies the body abundantly with minerals.

URINARY SYSTEM – THE EXCRETER

The urinary system excretes water, toxic waste and excess salt in order to maintain water and regulate the acid base of the body.

CHAPTER 3

Disease, Dismantling and Devastation

Our internal ecosystem essentially needs a diversity of beneficial organisms. Our gut microbiome is perhaps our greatest health asset. The gut microbiota harbors a complex community of over 100 trillion cells influencing physiology, metabolism, nutrition, immune function, vital organs and cognition. The delicate balance of this complex community can be disrupted by quality and quantity of water, poor nutrition and environmental sensitivities which may diminish beneficial organisms and create pathogens to overpopulate, affecting the whole body. We seem to already acknowledge the external ecosystem; I believe it is time we acknowledge our own ecosystem internally as individuals.

There are three major factors that contribute to why the human body has symptoms, detection and progression of sickness, illness and disease. They are below:

Malabsorption occurs when individuals are unable

to absorb nutrients from their food, such as carbohydrates, fats, minerals, proteins or vitamins.

Stress is a feeling of an emotional, physical and mental whole-body tension. Stress is your body's reaction to a command, challenge or change. Stress can come from a thought, internal health afflictions, external experiences with people and the environments you remain in and the environmental exposures. Including psychological trauma, addictions, behavior patterns and disorders.

Exposure to Toxins/Impurities everything you absorb through your skin, inhale through your nose and mouth, recreational participating and indulging. Including the inability to not release toxic accumulation of impurities from the whole body that ends up recycling and reabsorbing creating distress in the whole body. Allowing and not addressing these three major factors in the whole-body results in disease, dismantling of vital organs and body parts, which results in more stress and devastation of the whole body.

You are probably worrying, afraid and concerned about hereditary, genetics and deficiency. I understand. There is hope!

Are you interested in knowing which of these distinct systems addresses all three major factors listed above and gives your whole body an opportunity to cleanse, eliminate through releasing, restore and rebuild?

Hereditary does not completely determine what happens. Genetics study global inheritance and deficiencies are not your destiny!
- Wellness of Life

CHAPTER 4

Your Digestive System

The digestive system is the most undervalued system of the body. It is intricate and well made in order to give reinforcement to accomplish cleansing, elimination (releasing), restoration and rebuilding the body naturally.

EYES

Digestion begins with the eyes. The cells in our whole-body digest everything! Before we take our first bite of food, we take it in with our eyes. That's when the desire and craving begins. Let's think about TV commercials, billboards, technology devices and ads. Notice how when you have looked at the advertisement, your whole body responds and reacts. The cravings and desire occur even before you smell or taste what your eyes have just seen and been exposed to.

> *It is essential that I align every moment in order to manage myself*
> *so that what I see doesn't manipulate me.*
> - Wellness of Life

TONGUE/TASTE

Without flavor there would be no difference in taste. Flavorings, natural and artificial, add to the taste of food. Ask yourself, When preparing meat... without the seasoning would there be any flavor and satisfying taste? If you prepared plant based foods with the same seasoning could you enjoy the flavorful plant based food? Would you agree...It's about the flavor from seasoning?

Tongue – where primary taste is detected.

Salty and Sweet – front of tongue

Sour – sides of tongue

Bitter – back of your tongue

Umami (savory) – middle of tongue

This is so insightful. Sensory of taste happens... Before we even chew and swallow, the body is identifying how it needs to prepare itself in order to digest, receive proper absorption and protect the whole body.

NOSE

Smell receptors are the upper nasal passage nerve receptors that send information to the brain. What we smell is another factor in why cravings are demanding. Smell receptors are sensitive, sending messages to the brain and the brain reaction can be impulsive. Impulsive eating is different from compulsive emotional eating.

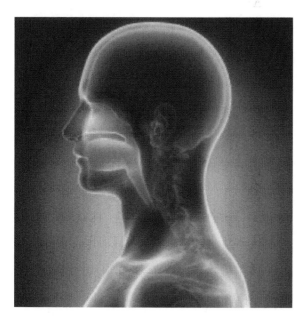

Impulsive eating is without thought. Compulsive emotional eating is premeditated. Example: Stating or telling yourself, you are an emotional eater before you eat. The goal is to have a healthy relationship with food.

PERMISSION...QUESTIONS TO ASK

YOURSELF:

Do you eat based on an impulsive reaction to a thought or smell?

Do you eat based on stress rather than address what is causing your stress?

Where do you think your stress comes from?

What are you stressed about at that moment?

In that moment are you... Board, Tired, or Thirsty?

Stress can be a positive kind request or negative demands you make of yourself. Maybe some people are not stressed because they don't allow demands from themselves or others. And if so, permission is granted to pause... Or I say bookmark, in order to listen, address, give and receive as you welcome that precious moment in time to process. Identifying the cause of stress. Therefore, creating healthier choices and decisions for the next meal. One meal at a time, each day. You have the opportunity to do better with each craving before you prepare or choose a meal to eat. Healthy relationship with food starts before we put it in our mouth.

> *Time is precious. Don't allow one moment to devastate your whole day... defeat your month and year... or demolish your dreams!*
> - Wellness of Life

MOUTH

Chewing is important. Chew, chew and chew. It allows the secretion of billions of good bacteria and enzymes to break down your food for digestion and attack bad bacteria.

Chewing is the body's first line of defense against bad bacteria, and pathogen invaders to be destroyed before swallowing. It will not allow bacteria overpopulation, as it protects your whole body before you even swallow. So if we are what we eat, we need to encourage ourselves to make a good decision before we prepare the food or place food in our mouths and chew.

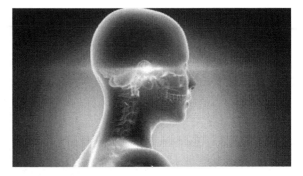

Chewing not only helps with breaking your food down for absorption on a cellular level. Chewing also activates the mechanical digestive system to function at its maximum capacity, stimulating peristalsis, allowing your large intestines (colon) to have a bowel movement, in order to release what no longer serves the body.

PERMISSION... QUESTIONS TO ASK YOURSELF:

Before you eat your food, Does this benefit and serve my whole body?

How do I want to feel after eating this meal?

How do I want to feel in the morning?

We need to have a healthy conversation about food to ourselves, not label ourselves emotional eaters. Eating whole food in season and real food is necessary for maximizing absorption to turn our food nutrients into energy and not slow down digestion, which can create putrefaction and stagnation in the whole body.

ESOPHAGUS

The esophagus lubricates and transports food to serve to the stomach.

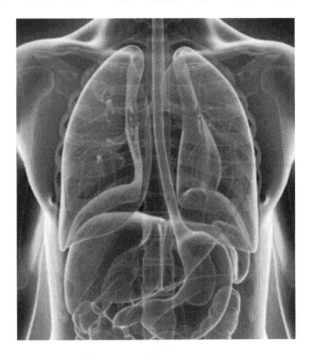

STOMACH

The stomach is a food reservoir for preliminary digestion. Some parts of the body are designed to be acidic to protect and prevent the body from pathogens and infection. The stomach does not just empty food all at once. The stomach is mechanically designed with HCL, pepsin, and gastric lipase to break down what the individual has swallowed before the food transitions to the small intestine for absorption.

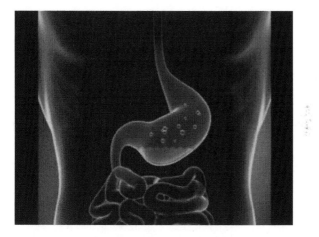

LIVER

The liver bile neutralizes stomach acid for absorption, filters impurities, cleanses blood, digests fats, proteins and carbohydrates. The hepatic portal vein drains the gastrointestinal tract. Bowel movements are mandatory, Because all systems release into the colon, your whole body is reabsorbing the accumulation of putrefaction and impurities back into the blood supply, overwhelming the liver when you don't have a healthy bowel movement and release.

Our liver processes everything we emotionally feel, exposure to what we give the body, and what we don't physically release. Learn to love and support your liver; it is a crucial, vital organ we cannot live without helping the whole body. The liver also supports the endocrine system. It regulates the hormones that can affect emotions.

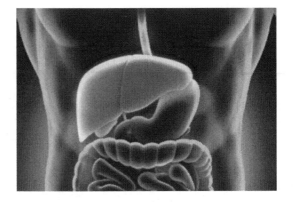

PERMISSION...ASK YOURSELF THIS QUESTION:

Do you often wonder about liver dysfunction, storing fat in the tissues of your body, mood swings, hormonal imbalance, or being emotional?

KIDNEYS

The kidneys' primary function is maintaining the water balance and keeping the acid, electrolytes,

26

sugar and protein balanced. Here is another essential vital organ to value for our whole bodies on a cellular level to function better.

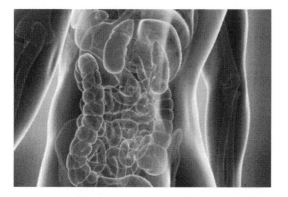

We have another reinforcement that we need to internally support us. Be kind to your kidneys; they, too... or should I say, they two are vital organs.

PANCREAS

The pancreas neutralizes stomach acid and regulates blood sugar. It helps the digestive system produce enzymes, so the enzymes can help break down our food for proper digestion and for regulating blood sugar. Regulating blood sugar can be complicated for some individuals. It is also the reason there are so many factors that can affect an individual's blood sugar imbalance.

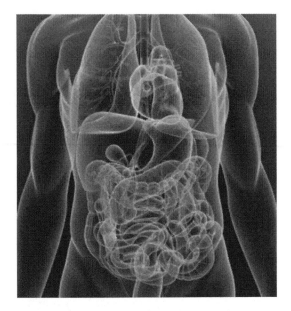

You don't have to have diabetes for blood sugar to be affected; some factors include what you eat, when you don't eat, waiting too long to eat, absorption, dehydration, stress, and constipation, Your blood sugar meridian is in your *Colon*.

We never used to hear about pancreatic cancer. Research has determined that under 200,000 cases of pancreatic cancer per year is rare. That's 1 million in five years. Rare? So if this is rare, explore the numbers on the other types of cancer that are above what research calls "Rare"!

SMALL INTESTINE

The small intestine has a big responsibility. Approximately 20 feet in length, Ninety percent absorption of water, minerals, food and nutrients should happen here. There are potentially a few billion good bacteria in the small intestine. However, malabsorption, constipation and stress can potentially create a storage of 10-20 pounds of accumulated waste and impurities in the small intestine compromising absorption and damaging the villi. The feeling of bloating and gas normally is associated with how the small intestines are functioning.

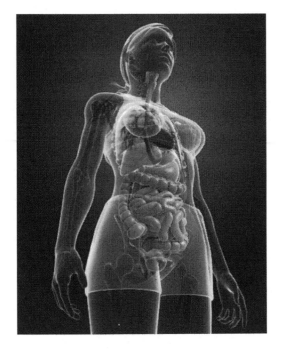

PERMISSION...ASK YOURSELF:

Do you suffer from issues of Poor Absorption-breaking down food, Anxiety, Gas, Bloating, Skin, Hair and Nail issues, Vitamin and Mineral Deficiencies, Appetite and Weight Issues, Microorganisms, Candida, H Pylori-stomach issues, Crohn's, Celiac disease, Leaky Gut, Sibo, GERD, and Inflammation?

LARGE INTESTINE (THE COLON)

The large intestine (colon) has the answers. It is one of the most important organs in the body and digestive system. A healthy functioning *Colon* supports the digestive system, and the whole body. Helping to address the three major factors of illness, sickness and disease. Malabsorption, stress, and accumulation of toxic, putrefied impurities affecting the health and wellness of the whole body.

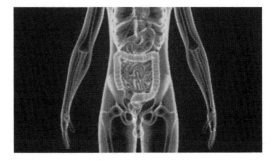

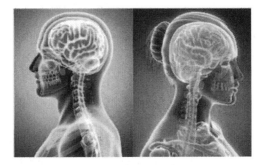

The *Colon* is approximately 5 to 5 1/2 feet long, can contain 10-40 pounds of waste and can have an accumulation of 3-4 pounds of bad bacteria. A substantial amount, as much as 70% of your immune system, is in your *Colon*. Trillions of good bacteria are in your *Colon*, ready to fight for your body like loyal soldiers. Ready to fight and destroy the bad bacteria invaders and create a thriving internal homeostasis community.

All systems of the whole body release into the *Colon*. The meridian system of the whole body also flows through the *Colon*. It is a distribution of our blood supply and body fluids throughout the body. The meridian system looks like a giant web network. This pathway supplies vital energy or sluggish stagnation. What pathway are you choosing?

The *Colon* and the brain are connected bio-chemically and physically, with the vagus nerve The vagus nerve runs from the brain through the face and thorax to the abdomen. It is a mixed nerve that contains parasympathetic fibres. The most important function of the vagus nerve is bringing information about the inner organs, such as the gut, liver, heart, lungs to the brain. This suggests the connection of the *Colon*, and vital organs are major sources of sensory information to the brain.

An astonishing 90% of your neurotransmitters are in your *Colon*. Neurotransmitters such as epinephrine, norepinephrine, serotonin and dopamine play a major role in controlling and maintaining emotions, nutrient absorption, blood flow, gut microbiome, and a boosted immune system for the whole body. Neurotransmitters communicate information to the nervous system for the brain to communicate throughout the whole body. Now 90% of our neurotransmitters are in our large intestine (colon) and we only use roughly 10%-15% of our brain.

Here are some brief descriptions of chemicals produced, released in the *Colon* and effects.

Endorphins – Stress and Pain trigger, the interaction with the opiate receptors in the brain. Higher levels help reduce our perception of pain, creating the ability to feel less pain and negative effects of both. A feeling of positivity and euphoria.

Serotonin – Is produced both in the brain and in the colon, which contributes to feelings of happiness and regulates sleep and alertness.There is a powerful link between anxiety, depression and digestion problems.

Dopamine – Plays a vital role in the feeling of happiness. In addition to our mood, movement, memory, and focus. High levels of dopamine create us to seek and possibly repeat pleasurable activities, while low levels can affect physical and psychological concerns. regulate emotions, memory, cravings, sensitivity to pain, and sleep patterns.

Glutamate – Normal levels play an important role

in learning. High levels can create insomnia, low energy and ADHD symptoms like inability to focus,

Norepinephrine and Epinephrine – Low levels are linked to fibromyalgia, migraines, hypoglycemia, and restless legs. Norepinephrine and Epinephrine are very similar neurotransmitters and hormones. While epinephrine has slightly more of an effect on your heart, norepinephrine has more of an effect on your blood vessels. Both play a role in your body's natural fight-or-flight response to stress.

GABA (gamma-aminobutyric acid) – Helps burn fat, lower blood pressure, and improve sleep. Low levels contribute to chronic pain and PMS.

PERMISSION...QUESTIONS TO ASK YOURSELF:

What do we use more of... 90% or 10%? Go with your gut when you answer.

However, is your gut healthy enough to make a clear decision?

Which one would you agree is the first and second brain?

Consider this...(based on 30 days in a month) If you are eating three meals per day, seven days per week, four weeks per month, that amounts to 84 meals a month, not including snacks. Now, take that number and subtract the number of bowel movements you are having.

For example, 84 meals per month, if you are having one bowel movement per day that is 28 per month. 84 meals minus 28 bowel movements equals 56 meals not released in 30 days.

In a month, having 2-3 bowel movements represents 60-90 bowel movements. Eat a meal and release a meal. The body should be preparing for the current meal you are chewing and transitioning and releasing the previous meal. Based on this example... How many bowel movements behind are you?

Infants are on mothers milk or formula and still have a full stool. Toddlers eat a meal and release a meal. As we become adults, why should this change. After surgery a bowel movement is required. The bowel movement is a indicator the body is functioning properly. So, if we are not having bowel regularity, Is our body function properly?

PERMISSION TO ASK...

Do you think you have a healthy functioning Colon?

How many bowel movements are you having daily?

Do you have Anxiety, Depression, Negative attitude, Cravings, or Addictions?

Do you suffer from Constipation, IBS, Colitis, Crohns and Diverticulitis flare-ups?

CHAPTER 5

The Best Offense is Our Defense Colon Hydrotherapy

COLON HYDROTHERAPY

Colon hydrotherapy is hydration supporting the whole body through cleansing the colon. Colon hydrotherapy is a safe, effective, gentle infusion of purified water into the rectum by way of a sterile rectal-disposable speculum. You lay comfortably on your left side. The process involves two disposable separate lines—water in, waste out—to prevent any possible contamination. This 30-45-minute session (duration may vary based on individual and complexity) The internal bath that helps hydrate the whole body, and the colon. Cleansing the colon, digestive system and whole body of toxins, impurities, gas and putrefaction of accumulated fecal matter during the consistent irrigation.

The FDA registered (closed system) allows excess waste to be eliminated through the disposable tube, the view tube and out the drain line without odor.

The colon is a muscle. Using the instrument in this way is like taking your colon to the gym. An internal workout. The instrument retrains and strengthens the peristalsis, the wave-like contractions, the urge you feel prior to having a bowel movement. Restoring the peristalsis responsiveness.

As adults, it is crucial to retrain the peristalsis. This so important because as children, teenagers and adult behavior... certain individuals have trained this muscle to hold, stop and not go. Delaying their bowel movements based on environment, timing and shame. Training the colon to become sluggish and unresponsive by not honoring the urge.

Colon Hydrotherapy brings back remembrance of what the body needs to do in order to obtain and sustain homeostasis.

Homeostasis is the property of cells, tissues, and organisms that allows the maintenance and regulation of internal stability.

The purpose of the instrument is to hydrate the whole body and colon, soften the accumulation of feces, irrigate the colon for elimination, and release what no longer serves our bodies.

Throughout and after the procedure, Wellness of Life clinical research is conducted and based on the condition of the individual's colon and digestive system after 3-5 or up to 12 sessions

(frequency varies based on individual and complexity) the result was more frequent regularity and healthier bowel movements, boosted immune system, mental clarity, less internal digestive disruption, reduced inflammation and cravings. Less weight issues, mood swings, anxiety, depression and drug addiction.

There is no other therapy in the world that uses pure water to hydrate the whole body, cleansing the colon, digestive system, and all systems of the body, eliminating impurities and supporting the blood supply. Healthier bowel movements, nutrient absorption, and helps with addictions and drug rehabilitation. In addition the procedure helps to slow down the aging process by providing better water hydration, nutrient absorption on a cellular in order for the cells to function, and flourish. Eliminating what overwhelms the body and compromises the oxygen flow. The individual walks away feeling hydrated, clear, refreshed and lighter from Colon Hydrotherapy cleansing the mind, body and spirit...all within a duration of 30-45 minutes.

Everything else in our lives updates, advances, has

new versions and evolves, including phones, TVs, automobiles, housing, appliances, technology, etc. Consider embracing the updated evolution of the enema—Colon Hydrotherapy.

The mucosa lining of the colon is what prevents the bad bacteria from entering into the tissue of the body. When the bad bacteria and impurities permeate the mucosal lining and tissues of the body, the pathogens enter into the bloodstream, allowing potential infections, illness and disease to occur. There is a strategy to cleanse the whole body with ease and it starts with cleansing the colon!

SHARED TESTIMONIALS ABOUT WELLNESS OF LIFE

Angela and her gift of colon hydrotherapy changed my life. Angela's motto "everything with love" is evident as she lights the path on your journey to health.

In 2018 a lump formed on my thyroid and my doctor recommended an ultrasound. The ultrasound showed a rather large nodule. I had a biopsy and the results were benign. The recommendation was to immediately remove the thyroid even though all my blood tests showed the thyroid was functioning perfectly. The pressure to remove the thyroid and start life-time medication was immense. Over the next year, I had five additional ultrasounds on my thyroid, saw a ENT, an endocrinologist, had an endoscopy and tried a variety of thyroid support medications. Nothing helped and they could find no reason my thyroid had a nodule. At every visit there was a recommendation for removal of the organ and medication.

I had seen Angela for colon hydrotherapy a few years ago and loved it. In complete desperation for answers I made an appointment for colon hydrotherapy. Over a course of a few months my heath has been restored. I believe my thyroid nodule was a sign of my weakened gut health and colon hydrotherapy restored that health. The nodule is gone and my energy, optimism and zest for life has returned. I am so grateful.

~ JL, Sacramento

My beautiful daughter has been dealing with some chronic constipation since the day she entered this world 10/29/1996. Over these past 20 years we have been to 12 specialists in Sacramento, Walnut Creek, Livermore and Stanford Children's Hospital trying to treat her and find a cure. So many tests, x-rays, hospital visits, feelings of helplessness, frustration, prescriptions—but never a reason "why" this is happening. We have tried everything to treat the chronic constipation and nothing worked. I have chosen to not give her prescription medication because the side effects were so horrible I just couldn't put her through that and risk additional long term issues for her. She wasn't old enough to make decisions for her body and we had to do it for her. It was up to her parents to make choices for her and hope and pray they were the right choices. I am so thankful these medical issues were not life threatening or terminal—but they were definitely life altering issues. We came to Angela desperate for help and hoping these colon hydrotherapy sessions would help her. Angela was very understanding, caring and professional. Both my daughter and I were nervous and scared this might not help. After meeting with Angela and a few sessions we noticed an immediate difference. Right now my daughter is pretty much symptom free and she has NO pain. She is a completely different person and is doing things she hasn't been able to do because she NEVER felt well. As parents one of the worst things is to see your child in pain and suffering and you cannot help them. I am overwhelmed with so many emotions right now.

Thank you Angela...you are an ANGEL and a lifesaver! XOXO

~ A&C Cooper

THE BEST OFFENSE IS OUR DEFENSE COLON HYDROTHERAPY

Immediately upon entering the "Wellness of Life" space you feel safe. Undergoing colonic hydrotherapy and the steps necessary to make your life better are not an easy process mentally or physically. Angela and her associates are not only professional and knowledgeable but they are understanding and accepting. They give you the tools you need to make your life better without being aggressive or judgmental. I felt immediately safe and secure to proceed with my steps towards wellness. I have had digestive problems for as long as I can remember. The most severe of the symptoms started about 5 years ago. In the past 5 years I have seen a plethora of doctors representing all natures of medicine. While they all gave me little steps towards progress I still found myself in a state of hopelessness. I was fatigued to the point of disability, could not eat without fear of discomfort and suffered random attacks of pain in my lower abdomen. As my last and final effort I went to see Angela at Wellness of Life. I think the tone and nature of this testimonial should speak for how I have improved. With each session I literally feel the life flow back into me. Seeing the waste that exits my body is physical evidence of why I felt so awful and why colon health is so vital. I am so thankful that I purged myself of this toxicity at such a young age (early 20s) because I cannot imagine how things could have been had I not. I am grateful to Angela and Wellness of Life for my newfound energy and for my future health. I sincerely hope that more people open their minds to the importance of colon health and overall wellness and insist that they start their journey at Wellness of Life."

~ Anonymous Client. April 2008

I highly recommend colon hydrotherapy sessions with Angela Harris at Wellness of Life. She is very professional, extremely knowledgeable and clearly cares about her clients well being. I have scheduled regular sessions with Angela since March 2007 and now my whole family enjoys the benefits of this important health care choice. I had experienced difficulties getting pregnant, despite 18 months of my husband and I trying to conceive. I was nervous and hesitant about trying colon hydrotherapy but Angela's experienced and attentive manner put me at ease immediately. After 1 month of colon hydrotherapy sessions with Angela, I felt more hydrated and less weary. I followed Angela's liver flush advice and continued with regular sessions and shortly discovered I was pregnant! I know that my sessions with Angela played a major role in my healthy pregnancy as I noticed that my overall nausea, swelling and fatigue was significantly less than when I was pregnant with my first child ten years ago. I have more energy, more control over sugar cravings and significantly less moodiness. My 9-year old daughter Maddie had suffered from abdominal pain and gas since she was an infant. Several different doctors had told me that she suffered from constipation because of a "slow moving gut" but none of their recommendations provided long-term relief. When my daughter's pain increased to the point she was missing 1-2 days of school each month and could no longer regularly participate in sports, I brought her to Angela. After one colon hydrotherapy session and by continuing to follow Angela's dietary advice, my daughter's painful stomach episodes have all but disappeared. I am so grateful that I found Angela and for the important role she plays in my family's good health and nutrition. Her services are worth every cent.

~ K.V.

———

"I would like to commend you for the wonderful job that you've been doing because you are saving lives. You saved mine. You have changed my life entirely. I was stressed, tired, depressed, and felt heavy, but now, none of that. I am so happy right now. I feel like a whole new person since I received my first colon cleansed, which was done over a week ago. I used to drink and smoke every day, but I haven't done either one since then...not even once. I feel so much better, physically and emotionally, and my skin has cleared a lot. I love it! I've been drinking plenty of water and exercising. Now, I wake up every morning feeling so alive, alert, and full of energy. Honestly, my first visit, I was really nervous because I didn't know what to expect, but you've made me feel very comfortable and NO PAIN. Thank you! It's been such a great experience. I've been telling my family and friends about this and referred you to them. You are amazing and I think everyone should see a colonist like you. Keep up the great work and I'll be seeing you again."

~ *M.T. Elk Grove, CA*

"I first met Angela in 2010 when I was diagnosed with a massive tumor in my brain. I was 23 at the time and decided on a natural path of healing. From the first time I spoke with Angela we had a powerful connection. I could feel in my bones that it was divine orchestration and that she was going to help me heal myself. I knew she was going to change my life. She changed my perspective on how we get sick in the first place and how we heal. She helped me to let go of the fear and to trust in the wisdom of my body. I had 3 colonics a week with her for about 4 months straight and went through her entire detox program. I had countless breakthroughs and could tangibly feel my body healing itself. It was a very

48

intense process of physical and emotional purging but I felt so supported by her.

Angela is a rare and special person. She has a soothing presence and very powerful healing gifts. Working with her though was one of the most spiritual experiences of my life. She helped me to connect. To tap into my power to heal myself. The sacred space she creates helped me to engage my courage and willingness. She taught me how to listen to my body and trust in my process. In 6 months my tumor shrunk from a baseball to a dime size. I transformed my health and my life through colonics with Angela and I will be grateful to her forever. Ten years later I'm thriving more than ever and still singing her praises. Thank you so much, Angela, for creating Wellness of Life and offering these powerful healing therapies."

~ M.S

CHAPTER 6

Lymphatic System

THE LYMPHATIC SYSTEM

The lymph, which is fluid within the lymphatic system, stimulates, targets and destroys invading pathogens. The white blood cells are made in our bone marrow and stored in our blood and our lymphatic system. The lymphatic system is a circulatory system separate from the cardiovascular system that carries water, white blood cells, and other substances. It does not have red blood cells or platelets.

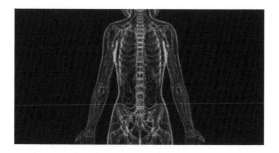

The lymphatic System is not the body's main carrier

of oxygen, lymph can move more slowly in the bloodstream, giving the white blood cells more time to find and attack bad bacteria invaders. The lymph vessels and capillaries drain away excess tissue fluid and does not return through the blood capillaries. Lymph fluid also absorbs protein from the tissue and returns it back to the bloodstream, then traps, and destroys bacteria, foreign substances and pathogens. Over 600 lymph nodes are prepared like troops, fighting and protecting you throughout your whole body.

> *Pay attention to your internal systems that protect and give you life, so you are able to prepare and manage the external stressors life reveals.*
> ~ Wellness of Life

CHAPTER 7

The Heart

The heart is an organ that pumps blood throughout the body all day long. Our hearts beat 100,000 times a day, pushing 5,000 gallons of blood through our bodies every 24 hours. The cardiovascular system consists of the heart, blood vessels and blood.

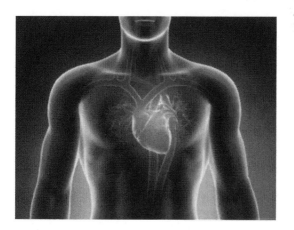

This system has three main functions:

1. Transport of nutrients throughout the whole body.
2. Promotion of oxygen to cells throughout the whole body.
3. Removal of metabolic wastes like carbon dioxide.

The whole body needs nutrients, oxygen and metabolic waste removed in order to survive and thrive. The physiology of the heart basically comes down to structure, electricity, provision and protection. Your heart has a rhythm, creating a heartbeat. And when it stops, everything about you stops!

This is why I believe in finding your Rhythm of Life! Your body controls your heart rate by the sympathetic and parasympathetic nervous systems, which have nerve endings in the heart. Neurotransmitters and hormones, such as epinephrine and norepinephrine circulate in the bloodstream. This triggers the heart rate to increase or decrease. Remember, 90% of our neurotransmitters are where?

Yes, the colon!

Are you familiar with fight or flight? The sympathetic and parasympathetic nervous systems are opposing forces that affect your heart rate. The sympathetic nervous system is triggered during stress or a need for increased cardiac output and sends signals to your heart to increase its rate. The parasympathetic system is active during periods of rest and sends signals to your heart to decrease its rate.

That is why I suggest lying on your left side during Colon Hydrotherapy. It is more relaxing in the parasympathetic state, which allows you to release the fight-or-flight mode. We can learn so much from the heart. Here is the best part!

Heart cancer is almost unheard of. Why do you think that is? Perhaps one of the reasons is the cells in the heart rarely divide! When there is division it weakens the whole structure and stability of the cells.

Our body cells divide when unhealthy. Like mindsets, families, communities and world issues. Because the cause is division, this may create a risk of cancerous cell growth. The negative begins to infiltrate, making way for illness, disease, bacteria, pathogens, and negative thoughts, words and actions. Unity is joined as a whole union.

Perhaps now you understand why holistic—looking at all aspects of an individual— the essence of Whole Body Health and Wellness with Ease not just focusing on the division of disease.

The opposite to this opposition would be opportunity for consistent positivity, cleansing, elimination, releasing, restoration, reconciliation, rebuilding relationships, emotional support, and creating a healthy belief system to encourage your mindset.

> *What is in your heart comes out in your words and actions. -*
> Wellness of Life

CHAPTER 8

There is Hope!

As you wake up each day, do you realize the magnificent miracle of life? How the body has the natural ability to protect itself even from us, and the potential to rebuild for survival one moment at a time. Shall we look at what the body is capable of doing?

The Intestines rebuild the most highly regenerative organs in the human body, regenerating (rebuilding) its lining, called the epithelium, every five to seven days. Continual cell renewal allows the Epithelium – which is one of the four basic types of tissue, along with connective tissue, muscle tissue and nervous tissue. Epithelial tissues line the outer surfaces of organs and blood vessels throughout the body, as well as the inner surfaces of cavities in many internal organs. Allowing the body to withstand the disease, dismantling and devastation it suffers when it is not supported.

ARE YOU SUFFERING?

H Pylori stomach issues, Candida, Crohn's, Celiac disease, Leaky gut, Sibo, IBS, GERD, Colitis, Diverticulitis, Microorganisms, Impurities, and Inflammation?

The Stomach rebuilds itself by replacing its lining every three days. The peptides (chain of aminos) repair the mucus lining, which neutralizes the stomach acid to prevent damage.

The Skin rebuilds itself in 27- 30 days. Skin Care of the epidermis is important...assisting in cleansing, and moisturizing during this process.

DNA rebuilds itself by cells constantly being renewed, and rebuilt every two months. What you digest determines the outcome of the cell structure. Remember, we digest everything.

The Liver rebuilds itself in six weeks. Reestablishing what supports detox and digestion.

Blood Supply rebuilds itself in four months. Having a full rotation every 60 seconds.

Old bones rebuild cells, and are replaced with new bone tissue within two-three months. The skeletal is rebuilt in 10 years.

New Cells rebuild every seven to ten years years.

Wellness of Life is committed to the cause... hope has already been given and provided to our whole body for us.

Consider what the whole body is capable of doing when provided with the resources, tools and wellness coaching committed to compiling a specific strategy with you. The daily assignment of contribution, educating and helping individuals live wellness of life.

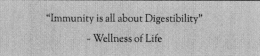

"Immunity is all about Digestibility"

~ Wellness of Life

CHAPTER 9

The Power of Releasing the Past

Decades of study—showed the type of relationship an individual had with his or her parents had an effect on their health in midlife. In some cases, this included significant health risks such as heart disease, cancer, hypertension, ulcers and alcohol abuse.

In all aspects of life, an individual can experience emotional, physical, mental and spiritual issues that could potentially affect every system, cell, brain and muscle in his or her whole body.

Wellness of Life conducted over 20 years of evidence-based clinical study that showed individuals released past and present emotions, mental and physical afflictions, and profound discovery about themselves, maturity and growth through verbally expressed stories, heightened positive results personally, family and career during Colon Hydrotherapy and Holistic Wellness Coaching. Individuals continued to have relief in the release. Various symptoms of health and wellness issues or concerns, throughout the repetitive series of Colon Hydrotherapy sessions seemed to go away. All sessions are based on the individual's health and wellness condition, needs and progress.

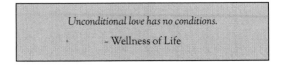

Unconditional love has no conditions.

- Wellness of Life

REAL-LIFE EXAMPLE

Here is an example, that might help you better understand what was mentioned earlier in this chapter.

A very special individual and I have had several conversations about the past at random times. Total empathy and compassion are the best words to describe the series of conversations, which in the past were sadness, serious and crazy hilarious. During one conversation, I told him that I could not speak for the other individuals. However, he had nothing to prove to me and I understood.

Another conversation with him went something like this: "In this moment," I said gently and very softly, "I forgive you. I release you and myself." He said, "Thank you," with a sigh of relief.

Sometimes we just need to sincerely talk about it, and after that it's time to release it. Meaning the thoughts of What if, and Why? no longer occupy space in my brain. That space is now free from whatever story I needed to tell myself to try to understand and justify it all. I know you're saying, She makes it sound so easy. Well, keep in mind I also said we had several prior conversations. Most of those conversations was reconnecting and connecting in order to realize the power of releasing. However, sometimes reconciliation happens first.

A helpful technique I use before having unpredictable conversations is I say, Kindly, We need to briefly talk. This conversation I don't want to have either. However, We need to have it. Then respectfully ask to arrange a convenient, realistic 15 minutes. If you have been thinking about it and it's been on your mind – prayerfully you know exactly what to say with Love.

People have their own stories they've lived and tell themselves. It warmed my heart to encourage him and show unconditional love has no conditions.

> *What we tell ourselves may not be the outcome.*
>
> *Love, trust and believe.*
>
> - Wellness of Life

ANOTHER REAL-LIFE EXAMPLE

Visiting, as I was traveling back home, I was standing in her living room wanting to reconcile. Prior to my arrival we'd exchanged phone conversations and sent text messages. Therefore, I had made arrangements. Repeating again now in person, I expressed to her I wanted to have a healthy relationship with her. I said, "I forgive you," and asked for forgiveness as well. She said, "What are you asking forgiveness for?" I said, "What is keeping our relationship apart, as we have said all we can say at this point? This individual felt I should do it her way and if I didn't, she would not accept it. Although I honor her with love and kindness. I approached it just as she requested.

Her way and still no reconciliation, no matter how much I communicated, argued, gave emotionally, financially or tried to resolve. Torn down again. Throughout my life I am truly thankful for all she has done for my family and I. However, at that moment, I had to make a conscious mental decision about her acceptance. Do I continue to have my spirit break or have a breakthrough? And realize it's between God and her.

When I walked away that day, I released myself. I hoped we would have agreed on the truth, solution and hugged that day, Instead I hugged and held on to the truth about that moment... until it set me free. Free from blaming myself for her thoughts, words and actions about me and towards me for many years! What a relief in the release!

The truth about the story you tell yourself is what the release is about and how it happens. Only the truth sets us free, not assumptions, others false accusations, lies and fairy tales.

PERMISSION...ASK YOURSELF THIS QUESTION:

Who and what do you need to release?

> *Everything is a relationship. Do your best to try to make it right and make sure it is healthy.*
> - Wellness of Life

CHAPTER 10

The Power of Belief

A clinical study showed that 94% of individuals believing in something greater than themselves contributed to their healing. Also, 86% of co-laboring practicing physicians believe that spiritual well-being is a factor in an individual's health. What you tell yourself and what you believe matters.

We can change our minds and shift our mindsets, however, it's when we make a decision to believe that is when everything changes.

Wellness of Life research showed individuals are more willing to have faith in a program when they hear or see others getting results. The issue was encouraging the individual to trust and believe in the program long enough to see results for their self before they gave up. Due to past experienced programs, trends, and other approaches individuals were mentally defeated.

The individuals needed a mindset shift toward the

truth about their current healthcare condition, and a whole picture, realistic, holistic wellness strategy for their needs and goals. Their concern is there are so many trending programs to choose from and deciding which would be the best fit for the them. One that would work and be able to sustain with ease.

When a different holistic approach was used, the individuals felt safe, cared for and trusted they could share the matters of their hearts and their struggles. The reason, I believe they received results is because their concern about their life, habits, family, work and social schedule was addressed. This is necessary to know in order to help.

How do you create a wellness strategy without information that is true, realistic, relevant and relatable to an individual's needs and goals? Questions asked by the individual and answers replied back from the individual matter most. Listening is imperative.

When opposition occurred, it gave an opportunity to grow by looking at the situation from a holistic whole picture view, teaching individuals how to align, assess and alter opposition occurrences. Talking about course correction, solutions and a strategy not "if" it occurs, but "when" it does occur.

Reminder... Opposition is God and the universe looking at you and asking, Are you ready to grow? Based on how you handle the situation, you will know exactly where you are at spiritually, emotionally and mentally. Look forward to growing and going through rather than focusing on the opposition. How else are you able to assess your growth? During opposition is when the true essence of who you are is revealed.

PERMISSION...ASK YOURSELF THIS QUESTION:

Do you have love, acceptance, patience, forgiveness, empathy and compassion for yourself and others?

Therefore, you have to be given the situations and circumstances for training, practice and testing in order to see your response or reaction, and determine what you have in your heart, mind and the depth of your essence that is within you.

Remember, when things are positive in your mind, behavior is easy to manage. Managing oneself during opposition reveals the character and integrity based on choices and decisions.

Insight...I would like to share as an Example:

My grandparents celebrated 68 years of marriage this year. I saw a lot in those years. My grandparents are very giving people. They believe in tradition and hard work. They taught me acceptance; work ethic; if you make a mistake, make it right; don't hold grudges and genuine healthy love wins. What I saw was both of them had the courage to be vulnerable. When challenged, they communicated their concerns with one another. Although the timing may have been off sometimes, they always remember how they took care of one another through hard times and divorce was not an option. Also, the task was accomplished by presenting a united front when addressing the family or a family member when necessary. We may not have liked tough conversations, nor did it feel good at times; however, connection and revealing conversations helped to teach us how to handle the discomfort and give all of us the opportunity to potentially grow.

Did they get it right all the time...who does? However, they never gave up and did not allow anything to destroy their bond and oneness. I witnessed a lot of forgiveness, acceptance, patience and love.

THE POWER OF BELIEF

Many times throughout my life I sat with my grandparents listening to their wisdom that helped my development. It was important for me to embrace and enjoy the foundation of family with tradition and memories that I still look forward to today.

In life, Always consider the source of information, to whom you are talking to, or reading, and the wisdom when you receive it.

> *When you shift your mindset, make sure you take belief with it.*
> *Your belief system regulates your mind.*
> *Be wise in what you decide to believe.*
> *~ Wellness of Life*

CHAPTER 11

Align, Apply and Activate

Alignment will help with the navigation of your life. When this happens the assignment becomes clear and can be accomplished effectively. Application is simply commitment to what you write. Think about writing your goals and visions down. Write down what matters to you, not a to-do list. Activation is very important for efficiency.

The analogy I like to use with my clients is, "Remember applying for a credit card? You have all that you need to apply! You already received it! You got it! However, until you activate it, it does not work." Two words, Work. Ethic. Go through it. Going through helps you to embrace what is happening, rather than questioning why it happened. No Shortcuts! Every moment of your journey is worth it.

YOU CAN'T GIVE...WHAT YOU DON'T HAVE!

My journey is Priceless because I paid the price...Sacrifice, Obedience, Consistency and Love...The willingness to endure the discomfort, and the tears of work ethic sweat! No one can take that from me! I paid the price and didn't give up! Therefore, I am grateful for it All.

Going around it is avoidance not addressing the matters of the heart.

Going under it is acting like everything is ok...a defeated sabotaging mindset.

Going above it is not holding yourself accountable...a superior entitled attitude.

There are wise people in the world. However, that does not mean they are applying the wisdom to their life or imparting wisdom. Going through the next challenging situation ensures the activated response will be different than a reaction to your life. If you don't go through opposition, how will you assess your emotional intelligence and celebrate the growth spurts?

For me, Aligning with God is loving myself. Trusting God and His faithfulness is having a healthy relationship of truth. Excited about the moment by moment, daily assignment he has for me. When I spend time in this relationship, I know how to have a healthy relationship with individuals. For me, this is self fulfilling.

> *The truth isn't always popular... However it is purposeful!*
> - Wellness of Life

How you treat others is a reflection of your heart and mind. Your emotional age, spiritual age and chronological age may all be different. Who you are and your thought process right now and the way you make choices and decisions perhaps may change in the future. If you are willing and choose to grow. In order to consider it growth, there must be change.Truth and wisdom knows the difference of change.

Seasons change, the year changes, time changes...what about you? Wellness of Life was able to see the difference in clients, in how they have grown and their belief system has strengthened their mindset. These clients released all aspects of their lives in phases. Research shows that healing requires an emotionally-charged setting, a confiding relationship and spirituality surrounding for the individual, in order for the potential healing process to have benchmarks of progress and breakthroughs!

Be a part of a person's breakthrough...not their breaking point!

- Wellness of Life

CHAPTER 12

Self-Care Requires Self-Compassion

Self-Care has two separate meanings. Self-care is the practice of what you should be doing for yourself to better yourself. Rather than the doing of your usual things, or a to-do list, be adventurous and go on a doting date with yourself. Plan and enjoy something you always wanted to do, create new moments and memories like connecting with nature. Take a nap and begin to dream again.

Self-Compassion helps you to have self-kindness about shortcomings and not ignore struggles that eventually turn into shame, self-criticism and self-sabotage. When you make a mistake—not if, but when—it takes real courage to make it right. Make an effort to make it right. Reconciliation is apart of restoration. If the other person does not receive, you have done your reasonable service, released yourself, and have closure for you. This helps with forgiveness for yourself and others.

Have tough conversations with yourself, expressing

the truth about *What* really happened in the situation. Not *Why*? The conversation may be hard for you, but necessary to have with yourself. The outcome may free you, so your mind is not held hostage by your actions and thoughts about yourself or others.

If you were to write a love letter to yourself, write two things you would tell yourself.

If you were to impart your wisdom to the younger you, what one thing would you tell yourself?

When were you the healthiest and most energetic in your life?

How do you assess yourself?

How do you see yourself in the world?

CONSCIOUSLY FOCUS, COMPETING COMPARISON AND HEALTHY COMPROMISING

Consciously focus on the next step. Don't focus on the finish line. Meaning, a determination to not allow distractions. If what you are trying to accomplish does not support the next step, then you've lost focus. You have to make the first step and move to gain steps of forward movement in order to create momentum. Everything before the finish line is essential.

You need to know what keeps you moving. Focus on WHAT motivates you. In our lifetime there will be more than one reason WHY!

Some people seem to know their WHY... When you understand WHAT motivates you, You will focus better. Because it will keep you excited about your WHY!

79

Keep moving and contribute your gifts, talents, skills and abilities. Competing Comparison causes you to focus on someone else's life. You lose your focus on what you need to be doing in order for you to stay focused on your own life consistently. Allow all your energy to flow into WHAT you are accomplishing. Remember, we have all that we need.

If you are the only one in the relationship who is compromising, limitations can occur, limiting your ability to move forward. Everything is a reciprocal relationship. Healthy compromise requires another person's effort, not just yours. Consciously focus on contribution and compensation automatically happens! You have to be available for abundance, not preoccupied with competing comparison and unhealthy compromise.

> Love gives and receives! We are taught to accept give and take!
> ~ Wellness of Life

CHAPTER 13

The Power of Water, Vitamins, and Trace Minerals

THE POWER OF WATER

Water is essential, it is a lubricant, regulates all functions in the body, dissolves and circulates. Water helps blood supply, brain power, releases impurities and waste.

Are you simply dehydrated? Let's see...

Colon Hydrotherapy revealed 95% of most individuals were dehydrated before their session. Amazingly 75% of most people are chronically dehydrated, And 50% of a persons thirst is often mistaken for hunger.

Mild dehydration will slow down one's bowel movements and metabolism.

One glass of water helps or can stop cravings and hunger.

Preliminary research indicates that 8-10 glasses of

water a day could help headaches, migraines, constipation, ease back and joint pain.

A mere 2% drop in body water can create lack of energy, short-term memory, trouble and difficulty focusing on the computer screen or a printed page.

Drinking five glasses of water daily decreases the risk of inflammation and stagnation, And contributes to obtaining homeostasis.

TRACE MINERALS BENEFIT THE WHOLE BODY.

Trace Minerals helps our body on a cellular level to Feel, Function and Flourish. The body needs minerals to absorb water, and food. Minerals are the super-charge for our bodies.

Trace minerals are important in the formation of the collagen found in bone, cartilage, and other connective tissues. It is also necessary for the formation of other connective tissues like elastin, which help maintain the integrity of the elastic quality of the body.

Recent experimental studies have shown that the benefits of trace minerals helps energy utilization, slowing down the aging process, creation and preservation of your bones. Also, assisting the part of the brain that dictates behavioral and emotional behaviors.

Trace mineral benefits include being able to serve as catalysts to vitamins within the cells of the human body, creating your cells to protect your body from bacteria, pathogens and viruses.

Most individuals suffer from trace mineral deficiency and severely lack the amount of trace minerals necessary to maintain and manage Whole Body Health and Wellness with Ease!

Research shows that fruits, vegetables, and grains grown on mineral deficient farms were compromising the absorption of the individual. No matter how much they ate.

Ninety percent of our absorption is in our Small Intestines. There has been a rapid increase of Malabsorption, which occurs when individuals are not able to absorb water, nutrients, and vitamins resulting in Malnutrition. Nutrients are Energy!

A mineral is an element or chemical compound that is normally crystalline and that has been formed as a result of the earth's physical structure and substance.

Minerals are naturally occurring substances that are essential for the Whole Body.

Minerals allow the body to receive proper absorption of water and food in order for our cells to receive the nutrients throughout our Whole body. Assisting with building bones, making hormones, metabolism, regulating your heartbeat, and supporting healthy muscles and brain function.

A vitamin is a chemical compound that is needed in measured amounts for the human body to work correctly. Vitamins are substances that are needed for normal cell function, growth, and development. Each vitamin adds value and serves an important role in the body. When you lack proper absorption of a certain vitamin, you may become deficient. Vitamin deficiency can cause health problems and may increase your risk of heart disease, cancer, and osteoporosis.

CHAPTER 14

Holistic Nutrition

Holistic nutrition focuses on a natural approach to a healthy diet and considers the individual as a whole, including all aspects of an individual's lifestyle. This natural approach incorporates emotional, spiritual and physical health to create a state of Whole body health and wellness with Ease.

Therefore, the individual's holistic nutrition program may vary based on goals, current healthcare needs, diagnosis and stage of illness.

HUNGER AND HEALTH

Everywhere an individual goes there is food and beverages. Several stores and restaurants exist on every street and in every environment, prepared and ready for purchase. Based on what you learned in previous chapters, do you understand what is happening internally? Hunger is a part of who we are. It's human nature to see food and want it.

However, once you taste it, it changes everything.

We want nutrient absorption, so our food can turn into energy and satisfy hunger, not empty calories in massive consumption turning into stagnation. Or a chemical to completely stop our hunger, which affects the digestive system and metabolism. Food is energy, not fuel. Fuel dissipates. We have teeth to chew food, releasing our own enzymes, and good bacteria for maximum absorption in order for our cells to receive the nutrients for our whole body to have energy.

After absorption, the mass still exists and needs to be released through our colon. Calories don't burn. A calorie is a measure of how much energy is in food. Some foods have lots of calories, some have a little. If there aren't enough calories in the food you eat, your body will not have the energy to function well. If there are too many calories, the extra will be stored as fat.

It's not about emotional eating or a food addiction, it's about having a healthy relationship with food. When you eat fruits and vegetables when in season, they are the most therapeutic for the whole body.

QUANTITY PORTION CONTROL

Based on research, a person can fill a small plate versus a large plate every meal for one year and could potentially lose nine pounds. What we eat, how we eat and who we eat with determines how well we chew our food, our stress level and whether we are taking time to enjoy our food. Take time to chew properly, then talk sensibly.

Have you noticed that at fine dining restaurants...you are given better quality of food, more time to eat and enjoy, and the portions are smaller.

Remember this... If you lack discipline on a meal, do better the next bite, next meal. Do not wait for the next day or week!

Nutrition Facts

16 servings per container
Serving size   1 Tbsp. (21g)

Amount per serving
Calories   60

% Daily Value*

Total Fat 0g	0%
Saturated Fat 0g	0%
Trans Fat 0g	
Cholesterol 0mg	0%
Sodium 0mg	0%
Total Carbohydrate 17g	6%
Dietary Fiber 0g	0%
Total Sugars 17g	
	34%†
Protein 0g	
Vitamin D 0mcg	0%
Calcium 0mg	0%
Iron 0mg	0%
Potassium 0mg	0%

* The % Daily Value (DV) tells you how much a nutrient in a serving of food contributes to a daily diet. 2,000 calories a day is used for general nutrition advice.
† One serving adds 17g of sugar to your diet and represents 34% of the Daily Value for Added Sugars.

NUTRITION FACTS

Labels on food products are telling you the serving size which is basically telling you the portions in the package.

The most important thing to remember about reading labels is the serving size, which is our "portion control" warning. The Nutrition Facts label above shows there are 16 servings in the container which means take the calories of 60 which represents 1 Tablespoon, multiply 60 by 16 which represents total calories in the whole package... 960 calories. Most people just read the calories, which may not represent the whole packaged product.

A good healthy simple start for portion control and proper food combining:

Try cooking less, eating on a smaller plate and chewing more.

Choose healthy foods you like and love.

Eat more fruits and vegetables than meat. There is more of a variety of fruits and vegetables than meat.

Rinse your meat, Soak your starches and grains, Wash your fruits and vegetables.

PROPER FOOD COMBINING

Main entrée meat and starch should not be eaten together if possible. Proper food combined is meat and vegetables or starch and vegetables. Maximizing better digestion, absorption and assisting bowel regularity in a timely manner. The chart below helps. This is based on proper food combining. When you do not properly combine your food, Food can take up to 8 hrs. to release from your stomach before it enters into the small intestines for absorption.

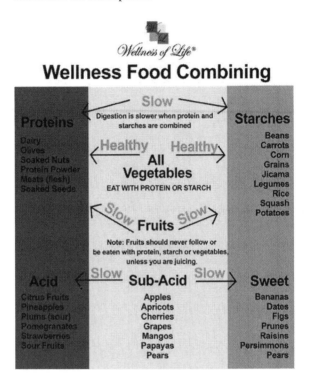

Transit Time to Intestines	
Water	0-10 Minutes
Juice	15-30 Minutes
Fruit	30-60 Minutes
Melons	30-60 Minutes
Wheatgrass Juice	60-90 Minutes
Most Vegetables	1-2 Hours
Grains and Beans	1-2 Hours
Dense Vegetable Protein (Nuts, Seeds, Avocados)	2-3 Hours
Cooked Meat and Fish	3-4 Hours
Shellfish	4-8 Hours
Any Improperly Combined Meal	8 Hours

Wellness of Life can help you develop a healthy relationship with food in any environment, using strategy and resources. Creating a belief system to fortify your mindset. Helping to find your rhythm of consistency and sustainability.

Preparation – We'll show you how to mentally prepare for changing your life for the better, based on all aspects being assessed...your personal life, career and social schedules.

Proactiveness – We'll help you stay motivated to

ensure results from your, Intervention to transition into Whole Body Wellness with Ease.

Prevention and Protection – We'll show you how to identify what is not benefiting your body currently, what is interfering, and how to stay focused on your goals. We teach you how to address diversion and release distractions.

> Food is energy not stagnation.
> ~ Wellness of Life

CHAPTER 15

FITNESS, WEIGHT MANAGEMENT AND ANTI-AGING

Fitness is important. It represents 10-20% of the whole-body health and wellness based on the individual. No matter what program you start—fitness or diet—most people lose the first 10 pounds in the first 2-3 weeks. Water, inches and inflammation. Individuals are not designed to eat what they want and apply fitness, which equals healthy. All aspects need to be addressed holistically for long-term sustainability.

Weight management is supported by cleansing the colon. It is a priority to help weight loss and maintain the weight that has been lost. The elimination of accumulated fecal and bad bacteria helps with a reduction of inches, less cravings, better absorption, assist liver support and boost metabolism.

The Liver can become overwhelmed with the exposure and reabsorption of what is not released. Trending fast, cleansing and nutrition suggestions have different effects on different individuals, reasons may not be compatible with your current diagnosis, health and wellness needs, which may create constipation and weight gain.

Due to constipation in the Colon (Large Intestine) not being addressed first. And not addressing the Small intestines, Can cause deficiencies and lack of absorption. The goal is to turn food into energy and fuel the cells in your body creating stamina and endurance.

By Cleansing and releasing the accumulation of fecal matter, impurities and bad bacteria out of your Large and Small Intestines you are able to jump start weight loss, maximize your metabolism, curb cravings, and feel more energy instantly or rest peacefully.

Anti-aging, There is no such thing as anti-aging. However, we can age gracefully by supporting our internal ecosystem. When you address the whole body holistically it includes providing resources and tools that address the internal health and wellness challenges, mindsets and beliefs. Internal stressors; Dehydration, Malabsorption, Malnutrition and Stress on the body can manifest noticeable externally aging appearances.

BODY IMAGE

Throughout our history there have been many different variations to what body type is in-style or is popular. Therefore, I tell young ladies, keep living your body type will be in style. It does not matter what body type you are. What matters is you are Healthy in All aspects of your life!

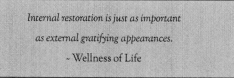

> *Internal restoration is just as important*
> *as external gratifying appearances.*
> ~ Wellness of Life

PERMISSION...ASK YOURSELF THIS QUESTION:

What footprint has been left in your internal ecosystem?

CHAPTER 16

Words Matter

The cells in our body feel, process and digest everything. Our thoughts, words, actions, experiences, environments and education affect us. The frequency and power of words and actions can now be evaluated and manifested.

If all the cells in your body digest words and thoughts, what are you feeding your body?

What have you told or telling yourself and your body about a situation, conversation or action?

What have you believed that was told to you and said about you?

What words and thoughts are you full of?

Just think! You are one moment away from what you choose to believe in order to grow. If this is the answer it would make common and social sense to use positive words. I know, you are thinking ... What about words of disappointments, distractions and adversity? My words of wisdom, love and kindness to you are...How are you able to ever know you have all that you need within you and it truly works... if you never get the opportunity to use the resources and tools during the opposition. Greatness is in you!

In order to grow spiritually, mentally, and emotionally... it requires internal courage and external focus. You can not overcome something you did not go through nor can you give what you don't have. What words can you tell yourself and believe in order to never give up?

QUESTION TO ASK YOURSELF:

Do you get your diploma, promotion or credentials *before*, *during* or *after* you go through the requirements in order to receive what you are focused on obtaining.

Before you speak, first self-assess and dip
your words in love, grace and mercy!
~ Wellness of Life

A MOMENT

Words do hurt! There will be pain and discomfort in our lives. However, just know...God keeps our tears. I believe my tears are kept in an extraordinary place.

When I realized God keeps my tears, I gave myself permission to cry when I needed to release. I asked God what was being revealed to me. His faithfulness. Do you know how close He is in order to catch and keep every single tear? Extremely Close! Supernatural Love.

CHAPTER 17

Healthy Relationships

Throughout the years of my life what I learned is the foundation of a healthy relationship is willingness, trustworthiness and unconditional love. Two individuals participating in the relationship and contributing to the relationship sets a structure for a healthy relationship. The relationship requires energy, effort and time.

If you connect and listen there is always a positive, revealing, reciprocal conversation happening of giving and receiving. The most important lesson I learned is to not allow any other negative distractions to take your focus off of the relationship. The negative represents anything that is not going to support the growth of the relationship.

Think of plants. If you wanted a plant to grow... Would you give that plant something that did not support its growth? Or think of a recipe that represents advice. Would you ask the wrong person for a recipe when you know they don't even know how to cook? Then you would be adding the wrong ingredients to the recipe and expecting amazing results. What do you think the finished product would be?

Therefore, the individuals have challenges in "the relationship" on top of managing the foundation of it. One or both individuals could be unhealthy, which can shift the structure of the relationship. The negative outside forces can influence and sabotage any relationship, including an individual in the relationship.

What is essential for me is having a relationship with God, with whom I align and trust in order to manage myself and determine the positive from the negative. Allow His spirit—the fruits of the spirit of love, joy, peace, patience, kindness, goodness, faithfulness, gentleness and self-control—to be the guiding force in the relationship. If you or other individuals are not contributing this spirit, ask yourself, Is this healthy?

Too much emphasis is put on "Apples don't fall far from the tree," rather than focusing on the fruits of the spirit and encouragement, And if you are a fruit inspector, make sure you are living the fruits of the spirit before determining whether someone else's fruit is positive or negative.

Meaning you cannot give what you don't have yourself. When a person says another person is not enough, others may say just enough, and someone else may say too much. It's just perception. Keep living! Allow and embrace the process of giving and receiving to happen. Please remember, do not mistake an individual's pruning process as a bad seed. Pruning has to happen in order to produce more fruit. MORE!

Think of "The Relationship" as the bank account of Love. If one person in the relationship was the only one working on the relationship and depositing love, while the other individual is not working on the relationship taking mental, physical, spiritual and emotional withdrawals ... Is this a healthy relationship?

The relationship requires both individuals to work together. Looking at the whole picture of the relationship. Connecting and communication is a healthy relationship. Finding the right time for both, to listen and express with the right tone and talk. Committing to both making love deposits and building the bank account of Love together. So when challenges happen and emotional withdrawals occur the bank account of Love is still sufficient... due to two people contributing to the account consistently, not just one.

EXPECTATIONS, ACCOUNTABILITY AND RESPONSIBILITY

A strong belief that something will happen or be the case in the future is an expectation. I believe you should not put false or mismanaged in front of the word expectations. Make a decision: false or mismanaged. If you make a mistake, do your best to make it right. Reconciliation allows restoration to occur for potential healing. The truth is as individuals, the relationship may not be the same. However, we need to be accountable and responsible.

There is a difference expressing I'm Sorry, I Apologize and Forgive me.

I'm sorry sometimes seems to be overused, I apologize, can be sincere, and forgive me shows accountability and responsibility.

It requires courage, commitment and consistency to do this, however, the result is priceless. To know you are trustworthy is a gift and contribution to the world. When you break commitments, you are cheating on yourself.

Through my life of shared parenting and being a single mom, I realized that teenagers number one priority is to get what they want. We as parents should not take it personally. It takes courage to stand firm in decisions consistently and not allow the manipulation of negotiating. I had to remind myself, everything else is noise. The commitment to provide for the family is based on the family structure or what is required to support the family responsibilities due to change.

The consistency is where I experienced the greatest benchmarks of parenting. My consistency created a culture of connection, and communication of truth which allowed the heartbreak moments to heal. I tell my children prior to tough conversations "You may not like what I am about to say, however, you can handle it. As well as I may not like what you are going to say to me, however, I will embrace it and handle it.

The Life skills I teach my children are learning what is beautiful inside of them. The gift that they have already been given by God, Healthy Relationships, How to connect and communicate with others, And most Important, Self-checking and assessing with Self-compassion.

My greatest service to my children is...

To see me have a relationship with God, Trust the wisdom through my experience and a healthy relationship with them and others. Dedicated to living, speaking and teaching *"Everything with Love"* consistently.

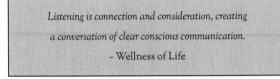

Listening is connection and consideration, creating a conversation of clear conscious communication.
~ Wellness of Life

INTERCONNECTION

How we live our lives during our lifetime needs connection. The interconnection can represent friends, family members, practitioners, and technology in this modern day society.

The need of connection is important for communication and support. This helps as a part of releasing as well. When people accept, show up and encourage you...It allows releasing negative notions...what no longer serves your whole body and giving yourself positive permission to be who you are designed to be with Ease!

COMMUNITY

Each individual's contribution to the world is

significant. In community there will be problem starters and problem solvers.

Through Togetherness we can share the difference to teach and learn from each other. Creating solutions, ideas, inspiration and encouragement to improve ourselves, family, friends, coworkers, social environments and community.

EXAMPLES

I have two siblings and I am the middle child. My older sibling and I are only 11 months apart and the same age for a little over a week. My younger sibling is five years younger. I have shared the older sister position and been the youngest for five years. I believe that, in essence, I can relate to all three of the positions. Therefore, It helps me with people interaction during interconnection.

One of my siblings has always been the mediator in the family and has tried to understand all sides during conflict. However this particular day of family strife she showed up for me on my behalf and stood up for me, supported me and encouraged me. I will never forget the connection of consideration and compassion she had for me that day. She just didn't hold space for me, she provided safety!

Friends can also be just as close as family, perhaps

107

feel like family at times. Being able to experience healthy friendships is necessary as individuals. Different healthy relationships are good. Because if one relationship is challenging, you have encouragement from other different healthy relationships. If you have one trustworthy person in your life that is good, two or three great, more than that you are lucky and blessed.

> *Your words and actions must align*
>
> *consistently in order to be trustworthy.*
>
> - Wellness of Life

Thank you for Time, Effort and Energy!
Truly Committed,
Wholeheartedly to Whole Body Wellness with
Ease!
"Everything with Love"
Angela Harris

CHAPTER 18

Resources, Tools and Support

Wellness of Life®
5120 J. Street #G
Sacramento, CA 95819
Online ordering:
www.wellnessoflifeproducts.com
Email: wellnessoflife@gmail.com
Clinic: www.wellnessoflife.com
Phone Number (916) 905-7743

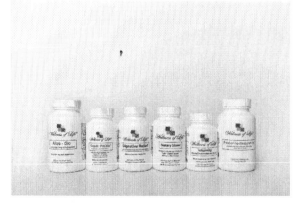

Internal Restoration Cleanse

3 Weeks / 21 Days

Package Quantity
Any 4 Supplements for $199.95

Includes:
Wellness Coaching and Instructions
Specific Daily Product Recommendation
Holistic Nutrition Recipes
Variations to Cleanse

Our products are dairy free, gluten free, soy free and vegetarian capsules.

Our commitment to quality, invested time in testing every single and multi-ingredient. The blends are carefully formulated to support specific systemic needs as well as to support overall health and wellness.

Our manufacturers/source has been producing quality supplements since 1979 in the USA.

Our shipping is packaged for preservation. Our recommendation for each professional product is initially taken as directed or guided with wellness coaching.

We believe in creating an effective program that is

realistic for you. We are all unique individuals evolving differently.

Our belief is there are three reasons illness and disease progress: malabsorption, toxins, the inability to release the impurities, and stress.

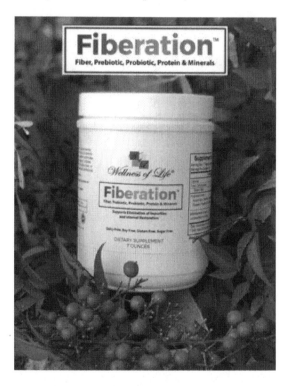

Fiberation™

A substantial sugar-free powder formula to help support whole body health and wellness with ease.

Add to juicing, make a smoothie, sprinkle on oatmeal or cereal, and you can even use for baking healthy snacks.

What makes this product supreme?

A good amount of **Fiberation™** is Protein, Fiber, Prebiotic, Probiotic, Omega Fatty Acids, Amino Acids and Minerals.

ENERGY

Satisfies Hunger and Promotes Bowel Regularity.

Helps maintain blood sugar, hormones, blood pressure, and cholesterol.

Helps infection and inflammation.

Helps absorb heavy metals, in order to release impurities.

Helps the bifidobacterium to colonize, sustain and over populate creating a community to protect and support your whole body wellness with ease.

Also, B complex vitamins and vitamin E, as well as minerals such as magnesium, potassium, and iron. Vitamin E is essential for healthy skin and bones. Potassium maintains nerve health and iron is a vital component of red blood cells (oxygen in – waste out) and many enzymes that affect our general metabolism.

Helps Cravings, Candida, Leaky Gut, H-Pylori, Crohn's, Sibo, IBS, GERD, Colitis, Diverticulitis, Hemorrhoids and Varicose Veins

CLEANSING PROGRAM

Taking ½ – 1 teaspoon of **Fiberation Powder™** added to water, juice, or smoothies daily to get enough natural fiber, protein, prebiotic, probiotics, and minerals. **Fiberation** helps your digestive system release by restoring, supporting and creating natural peristalsis movement in the bowel. If you are constipated and do not have at least one bowel movement daily, take 1-2 capsules of **Aloe-Go™** to promote bowel regularity. For Small Intestines, Inflammation, and Liver support 1-2 capsules of **Inturnity™** with these three products working together synergistically to aid your body's digestive system to eliminate properly and support Whole Body Wellness with Ease! Also, our **Super-Probio™** has changed the digestive system and the lives of many individuals, receiving results in 2-4 days.

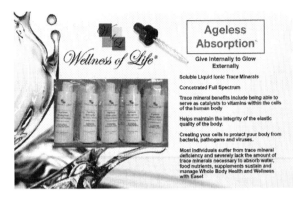

Ageless Absorption™

Better absorption, skin and beauty – Helps maintain the integrity of the elastic quality of the body, electrolytes/trace minerals for cell support -1-2 drops added to water or juice based on your body weight.

SPECIALIZED PRODUCTS

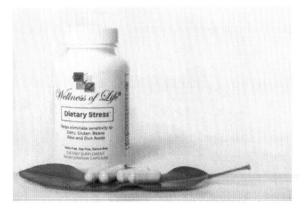

Dietary Stress™

Promotes digestive health and helps eliminate intolerances and sensitivities to dairy, gluten, beans, raw and rich foods, heartburn, congestion, and acid reflux. Supports the pancreas and helps regulate blood sugar, fluid retention and reduces candida. Breaks down fat, starch, lactose, and halts for better absorption. Amino acid for vegetarians. Also, Prebiotic and Probiotic.

.

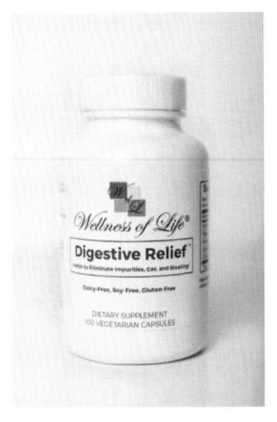

Digestive Relief ™

Digestive Relief has the ability to alleviate gas and bloating. It can promote digestive health and rescue. Helps eliminate food poisoning, impurities, reduce inflammation, helps mental stimulation, helps improves memory and provides cognitive boost, supports chelation and drug rehabilitation.

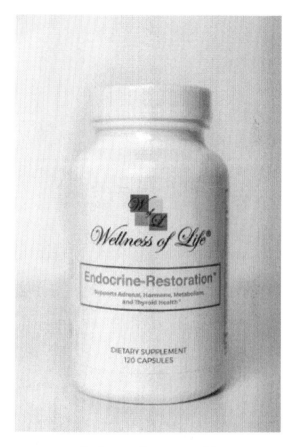

Endocrine Restoration™

Supports adrenals, thyroid, hormones, and
metabolism.
All about the Vitamin B's.

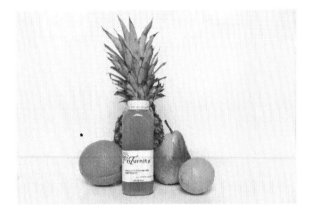

Wellness of Life has created
Inturnity Herbal Juice™

Ingredients: Orange, Lemon, Apple or Pear,
Pineapple, B-12, Nettle, Activated Charcoal, Apple
Cider Vinegar, Camu, Turmeric, Raw Honey

Flavors: Cayenne, Ginger, Mango/Jalapeño,
Peppermint, Watermelon (seasonal)

A strategy for individuals to turn toward a state of
well-being. Restoration and refining begins within,
allowing the body the opportunity to rebuild itself.

Cold-pressed juice infused with a blend of herbs
and supplements that have the natural ability to
substantially impact the health and wellness of the
individual. We believe by specifically targeting
digestive health it provides an exceptional

environment for absorption. Maximizes cleansing, better digestion, immune booster, supports the liver and lymph, and stimulates the circulatory system.

About the Author

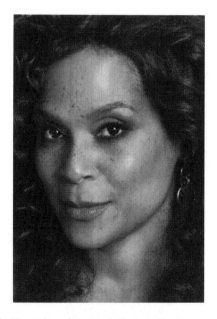

Angela Harris was born in Western Europe, raised in Anchorage, Alaska and replanted in Sacramento, California. The founder of Wellness of Life Internal Restoration Clinic, InTurnity Herbal Juice, and Wellness of Life Supplements, she's been a truly committed entrepreneur for over twenty years, serving and contributing to holistic health and wellness. Recently, Angela became an author and shares her knowledge in her first published book, Whole Body Wellness with Ease NOT Disease.

Her passion for healthcare began at nineteen while attending college and working at a holistic integrative medical / dental clinic—just a small town girl driven to make a profound positive difference in people's lives. Angela was given the opportunity to attend the American Academy of Environmental Medicine, where she became certified in Environmental Medicine specializing in food and chemical sensitivities, along with cognitive, behavioral reactions and environmental inhalant allergies. Through this experience, the essential need of colon hydrotherapy was revealed. She is an I-ACT member and National Board Certified Colon Hydrotherapist, Instructor and Educator of Anatomy / Physiology and Holistic Nutrition.

At her clinic, she implements Holistic Wellness coaching, educating and cleansing the mind, body, and spirit. Nutrition and dietary counseling are addressed to support the digestive system. During visits, an individualized Holistic Wellness Strategy assessment is created to transform her client's current health care into self care Whole Body Wellness with Ease!

Her continued education is dedicated to expanding her knowledge while maximizing her experience in Internal Restoration, Holistic Nutrition, and Holistic Psychology.

Angela's motto in life is "Everything with Love." She believes in interacting with people and finding that common thread of purpose. She enjoys sharing love, and laughter with her family and friends. Her hobbies are Aligning with God, connection and creativity, experiencing nature and traveling.

Made in the USA
San Bernardino, CA
28 June 2020